A Walk on the Dark Side

Paul Brookes

45 Years on Insulin

CONTENTS

Acknowledgements

To Barbara and Jennifer who between them, for many years, kept me going.
They have bailed me out of countless difficult situations.
To Leanne and Laura, my stepdaughters, who provided the casual, stress
free innocence that kept the family rattling along.
My typist Amy Rose, for deciphering my handwriting,
asking questions and probing my notes.

Preface

Insulin is not a cure for diabetes; it is a treatment, and an imperfect treatment at that. People with type 1 diabetes on insulin in particular are prone to fluctuations in blood glucose levels and also to complications arising from their condition. In many diseases other than diabetes, treatments are simply prescribed or carried out by a doctor. By contrast, in diabetes, although patients will receive help and advice about insulin treatment, day to day management of the condition with diet, exercise and insulin is largely up to the individual.

These aspects of life with diabetes are vividly described in this book by Paul Brookes. This is not a medical textbook, and should not be read as such; rather it is an individual and personal testament to a life with diabetes. Problems and events related to diabetes are described not from the clinical point of view but from direct experience. The initial diagnosis of diabetes and 45 years of living with the condition are colourfully laid out. The effect that one person's diabetes can have on others, and in particular close family members, are made clear.

In particular Paul describes the development and treatment of diabetic eye disease and the concern about the effect that diabetes can potentially have on eyesight. Above all, he shares his individual and person experiences of the bizarre world of severe hypoglycaemia, (where the blood glucose falls sufficiently to affect brain function) – with various often unpleasant or frightening effects and occasionally humorous consequences.

Peter Mansell
Consultant Physician
Department of Diabetes and Endocrinology
Nottingham University Hospitals
April 2011

Introduction

My next birthday is my 60th and I became a type 1 Diabetic when I was 15 years old. That's a fair number of years on a daily dose (now numerous doses) of insulin. Over the years I have had uncountable experiences to which many people have said "You should write that down", either because it was funny (depending on your sense of humour), perhaps medically intriguing, a footnote to other diabetics or just plain interesting.

I've read somewhere that long term use of insulin makes diabetics depressives. Either because of the chemical effects of insulin itself, or the downright slog of balancing up insulin with food and day to day life.

In my case, I'm a bit weird; insulin has made me look at my life from another angle. I'm not saying that the hypos I've had are not medically serious for me, but from another viewpoint, I've provided a few laughs for friends and relatives.

It's important to say, that most of the time I'm a well balanced, serious thinking person that can easily hold my own in most environments. Professionally I was an academic for over 30 years, being a maths teacher, then Head of Maths in a large comprehensive school. Then of course, as any long term type 1 diabetic knows, there is the frightening side and the downright hilarious side...

This is my life so far. The dates are a bit hit and miss. Hang on tight.

To
Barbara and Jennifer

Chapter One: 0 – 14 years old (or 1951 – 1965)

I was a very healthy lad. My dad was a carpenter, my mum a housewife, and my brother, four years older than me, a craftsman like my Dad. We lived in a council house in Chasetown, Staffordshire.

As most parents did in those days, we were kicked out to play during holiday time at 9 ish, after dad had set off to work on his bike so that we wouldn't get under foot. Mum was the boss.

We made bows and arrows out of the straight bits in hedgerows and put lethal steel tips on the arrows to kill anything at 50 paces if we could hit it. We made bombs out of weedkiller, charcoal and sugar, as you do. Soda siphons did the job. My cousin Peter was a bit older and provided the initial training.

Mrs Richards at the local model and hardware shop used to ask me when I went to buy the ingredients for bombs, whether I was making bombs. I said no, she looked hard at me, took my money, and everyone was happy. We did a bit of damage to the drainage pipes at the Pool (later called Chasewater), but survived to tell the tale.

When I was about 11, we went on our annual holiday, by coach as always, to Great Yarmouth. We met another family there and Robert (my brother) and myself played with a boy called Nigel. This had perhaps the most significant effect on the rest of my life. He was a very, very keen trainspotter.

From then on, inspired by Nigel I used to bike everywhere, miles and miles and miles to the steam depots of the Midlands. I think my Mum was as pleased as me. I went off at about 8 in the morning, with cheese and tomato ketchup sandwiches, some fruit cake and a flask, and didn't get back 'til dark, then off again the next day.

Just another independent, motivated, healthy schoolboy.

Cassius Clay v Sonny Liston, 25th May 1965

I can pinpoint the day. Amongst all my other activities, I was a good cross country runner and represented the county. I supported Walsall FC – the Sadlers. One particular day I went by coach to see them play at Colchester.

God, I was thirsty. I had a large bottle of pop with me, which I drank before our first coach stop, then had a hot cup of tea at the first stop, and bought some more pop. At the ground I seemed to be going to the loo a lot, and bought even more pop.

When I got home, I was feeling rough and really, really tired. Mum and Dad were out so I sat down to watch the boxing match that had filled the sporting world with such excitement. Cassius Clay (now calling himself Muhammed Ali) versus Sonny Liston. It was over quickly so, exhausted I slept.

In the morning I was off to the doctors with my mum – the following day to the hospital at Walsall, where they kept me in. A week later I left with my new glass syringe and some insulin.

I wasn't really phased by it all. My mum could handle anything and this rubbed off on me. Actually, to be more accurate, it went over her head. For the next 40 years until she died, she never really understood diabetes.

At a local cafe in Walsall after a hospital visit, mum ordered some food, but I couldn't have many chips, as she announced to the chap serving "He's diabetic you know." I was soon going to the hospital alone, but not really understanding what was happening. I got up at 6.30 to do quite a long paper round, I did a bit of running, played football for the school – so what was was the problem?

In those days, the only way to check your blood levels was to test the amount of carbohydrate in your urine. This meant collecting urine and with a dropper counting 5 drops of urine to 10 of water (I think) in a glass test tube, then adding to a tablet. The colour after 30 seconds of fizzing, gave you the result. Mine was always high, but so what, I felt ok.

Chapter Two: 15 – 26 years old (1966 – 1977)

I don't think I had a hypo during this period. Lots happened during this time, but nothing out of the ordinary. You wouldn't have known I was diabetic unless I told you. I had my insulin every day, (one injection in the morning) and went for an annual visit to the diabetic clinic, but it was more of an inconvenience than anything, particularly when I was at college.

I was quite a good model maker – usually plastic kits, which I did during my free time and continued doing when I started teaching. It was good nerve therapy, especially the big complicated Japanese steam locos. I had good eyesight and steady hands, which helped of course.

The years '66 to '77 went a bit like this:

a)   good GCE's

b)   and A-Levels

c)   girlfriend – she physically drained me

d)   Sussex University for B Ed

e)   another girl – got engaged. It didn't last. She was an Essex
      girl. Her father didn't like my Black Country dialect.

f)   started teaching maths at Quorn Rawlins Upper School near
      Loughborough. Played a lot of squash.Rented a room in a house
      with three young women. An experience.
      Drove a car and took the school minibus abroad – as you do.

g)   girlfriend – lots of parties

h)   walked the Pennine Way. Almost hypoed for the first time. I
      wondered what was going on, but clearly, something wasn't quite
      right.

Chapter Three: 26 – 38 years old (1977 – 1989)

This was the period when it all kicked off. I was promoted to Second in the Maths Department at Branston School and Community College in Lincolnshire. Barbara, my girlfriend (later my wife) followed me up some weeks later and we had a lovely cottage in Potterhanworth. I drove or biked to work every day.

I was very practical, doing a lot of major work on our cottage, in the garden, cutting hedges, restoring antique furniture, producing school plays. I took insulin every day, my urine carbohydrate levels had always run high, I felt 'as fit as a fiddle'.

Because of my physical activity during this period which involved working all day, building work many evenings, playing sports, I experienced my first hypo. Too long ago now to remember the details.

The Dr Scott incident

Now Dr Scott was nearing retirement and unfortunately only had one eye. He was well known for his almost lethal driving skills. He knew me as "the man who lives with a woman" Barbara and myself were not married at this time which didn't sit too well with him.

On this particular day I was at work, teaching maths to my not very able 5th form group (now known as year 11s) who were challenging my patience as usual.

I'd been playing 5-a-side the night before and was now aware that blood was leaking into my eye from above, so out came the tissues, but it wouldn't move the blood. I went to the Staff toilets to have a quick look, but there were no visible cuts. A quick call to Dr Scott followed and he said he thought he might know what it was and I should go home and lie down, which I did. I was now 29 years old.

Of course, I'd had a bleed in my right eye, and blood was swilling around. Dr Scott was not the sort of guy that suffered fools gladly, he was very matter of fact about life. He said that he had got me to be seen at Lincoln Eye Department and see what they could do (no laser back then) and failing this I could go down to Moorfields Eye Hospital in London where they had a laser. I think it was the only one in the UK at that time. He then added, "Fat lot of good it did me." Within two weeks, my left eye had bled as well.

First eye treatment

After my eyes had cleared I went to Lincoln, where the treatment was a bit scary. In essence, they gave me a local anaesthetic via a big needle, above and below the right eye into the bone. It really hurt. A young nurse, assisting the consultant and two staff nurses fainted and the consultant lost his temper with the nurse. Nevertheless I was put into a wheelchair (my senses were affected so I would fall over) and waited for the anaesthetic to work.

In these days the process was to use bright lights that were shone into the eye to pinpoint and coagulate the blood vessels. It didn't work.

Off I went to Moorfields Eye Hospital with Barbara. Evidently I had jumped a large queue to get there. It was pointed out to me that as money had been invested in my education, they needed to keep me going in order to get some return on the country's investment. I still think about the queue of older patients that were perhaps missing out.

I sat in a small corridor offshoot of a main corridor, with an inconspicuous door marked 'Laser'. A small suited gentleman walked past and asked to see the file I had been given. He said to hang on and he would do me himself. This was Mr Blach, the main consultant at the time. He had just returned from America where he'd been giving lectures at their eye clinics.

Eventually I sat in front of one of the now familiar eye inspection contraptions with Mr Blach sat opposite me. A lens was put into my left eye to help his aim. I gathered that it was a bit like playing space invaders with a laser gun. Just keep firing until you hit a burst blood vessel. My eye was getting uncomfortably warm.

He said he could see a couple of exposed nerves near the target area, so I asked what would happen if he hit one. "You'll know," was the brisk response.

Inevitably of course, my head shot back involuntarily and I fell off the stool. "Are you alright?" he enquired.

My left eye was now very hot and very painful, but it was now sealed, and an appointment was made for my right eye in two week's time. Unfortunately, the damage in my right eye was severe and the retina detached, leaving no chance of a surgical solution.

So back to work straight away, left eye working (I'm left handed!!) and right eye blind. It wasn't long before I realised that my night vision for driving was not great, with just one eye, and that being lasered. This was reinforced by our lodger Kit (another school teacher) who went into an uncontrollable screaming fit as I gave him a lift home one dark night through the Lincolnshire Wolds. Barbara talked me into not driving until my sight had recovered.

The mortified student incident

As Second in the Maths Department it was my job to mentor the maths students from the local college – writing their reports etc.

I walked into the staffroom one morning trying to find Mel, a maths teacher. Struggling to see much further than a few feet, I said to the maths student next to me, "Where's Mel?" He turned around quickly and said, "He's here. Are you blind or something?" Mel was sat right in front of me. The Head of Maths, who was nearby, put his arm around the student and walked him away, talking quietly into his ear.

From then on, the poor student was a nervous wreck every time he was near me. Of course, your best mate always takes a different angle. From then on Kit took any opportunity to bellow out, "Are you blind or summat?" Usually it was if I tripped over, or missed a goal being scored at Lincoln City – which didn't happen that often.

Mrs Baker's Theory

Mrs Baker lived just down the lane from our cottage. We were surrounded by fields and to get to our cottage you travelled along a minor road from Potterhanworth, took a farmers lane for 200 yards and then a hardcore lane for 100 yards. Quite isolated, but lovely.

Mrs Baker was the local cleaning lady. About five foot tall and almost as wide. Her husband was perhaps the same height, but very skinny. They drove a Reliant Robin. Deep meaningful conversations were difficult, but she liked her cigarettes.

When Barbara pointed out that I was diabetic and had to be careful with certain things, Mrs Baker showed her understanding of circulation problems very quickly, as she had a diabetic friend. She said that because diabetics had eaten too much sugar in the past, that after a while the sugar fell down their bodies, through their legs to their feet. There it went hard, so the diabetic had to have their feet cut off. Since then, at Christmas time I go a little cold when I see sugar pigs and trotters in the shop windows and say to myself, "No! Surely not!"

It was at this stage that I was hospitalised to try and get a good control of my blood sugars. Barbara was good in a crisis; you had to be brave or stupid to take her on if she was looking after your welfare.

On going into hospital Barbara remembers the Ward Sister being a bit like the Matron in the 'Carry On' films. Terror ruled the ward. Even the doctors did as they were told. Anyway, this Sister was being a bit stroppy with Barbara, so on the Sister's retreat to terrorise someone else, Barbara let everyone in the ward know that she was going to make an official complaint.

This resulted in all the patients, no matter how close to shedding their mortal coil they were, begging Barbara not to say anything as the Sister would heap her revenge on them all and no one would get out alive. Barbara agreed on a cessation of hostilities and a tactical withdrawal, provided no one saw this as a defeat.

Upon my paroled release a new regimen was in place. I took Insulin twice a day and kept tight control of my blood sugar levels. DIY blood kits were not available yet, so this was easier said than done.

Testing urine means that you can only get an idea of your carbohydrate levels after digestion of food. Consequently, if you had low blood sugar, you wouldn't know until sometime later. The wrong way round really.

Moorfields Eye Hospital – again

This was always a trek from Potterhanworth. The car was hard work for Barbara and so I nearly always went by train.

I was always impressed by the number of people working at Moorfields. To me there were more chiefs than indians – so service was quick and you felt confident. I always remember a group of people in white coats observing my consultant. I asked one what he did at Moorfields, and he said he was an American visitor, about to open an eye clinic in the US, and they had come to see how the experts did it.

Whilst this was encouraging, seeing patients in a far worse condition than me, in a strange way made me grateful. One girl I remember, perhaps about 18, almost blind and about to go blind, was sitting in a wheelchair next to her mother. She was full of the joys of spring, chatting to me and asking me about Integral Calculus (tough sums). I thought, "Shit, what am I grumbling about? I've still got my independence, I'm able to work and get out."

On return to work, the chaps were blown away by the colour of my wee. It was bright yellow. A dye had been injected into me to highlight the back of my eye so that photographs could be taken. The comments at the men's urinal were a combination of "err" and "bloody 'ell". Luckily enough it dissipated after a couple of days.

Low blood sugars and hypos at Potterhanworth

These don't come in any particular order, and I'm sure I've missed a lot out. These are the ones I remember for various reasons.

Elaine worked at Branston with me, and she and her boyfriend Martin, an RAF policeman, became very good friends. Unfortunately they split up and Martin came to live with Barbara and myself. One day Martin and myself went into Lincoln to collect and pay for a carpet and whilst Martin was fumbling with the carpet, I got out my cheque book and just stared at it. I couldn't remember how to write a cheque, or even sign my name. Martin didn't like to interfere, but had to.

Martin always saw us as the people who bailed him out, and so called Barbara "Mum" on occasions when he was being told off. On returning home, he delivered the line, "Dad's had a silly." It's one of the phrases that has stuck.

I am not a medical scientist, but the way I think it works on me is like this. The insulin reduces the blood sugar levels in your body. If there is too much insulin, it looks for more blood, with carbohydrate to work on. The last remaining part of your body with a considerable blood supply is your brain. Insulin then tries to work on this last reserve of blood.

The brain, being a wonderfully developed self protecting machine, then begins to switch off aspects of the brain to protect itself. This is why diabetics, whose blood sugar is falling, seem to be drunk, as facilities are shutting down. No different to the effects of alcohol on the brain. Eventually of course there is serious shutdown and a coma. This is the "Brookes theory".

How many diabetics out there have experienced low blood sugar where they can still function reasonably well, but rationality and social learning is the first to struggle and you appear to others to be in a daze? I have been able to slowly walk home with low blood sugar as walking is further down the physical/learning scale, than say talking.

Non diabetics don't usually understand the next bit. They say, if you feel that your blood sugar is falling, (for example pupils dilating and so brighter light) then take some glucose. Sounds fine.

The problem is, that by the time that you get to the level where a sense picks this up – it's too late. Powers of rationality and thinking are compromised. I can't even think a simple problem through. I continue to drift and slowly shut down.

One low blood sugar incident sits in my mind as nothing like it has happened before or since. Our cottage (well, 2 of a row of 6 really) was surrounded by fields, so no passing public, except the neighbours, who were at work. I think I may have been gardening and came to the front of the house where we had a lawn. I can only describe it as odd. I found myself, lying on the lawn, gyrating around in circles on my side. Occasionally I would roll onto my back with my legs doing cycling movements. I was in a kind of suspended trance, not getting any better or worse. I didn't have the strength or ability to stabilise myself and get up – not that I wanted to. It was bordering on being frightening. After perhaps fifteen minutes, I lay down quietly and slowly recovered. I think my liver must have secreted just enough glucose to feed and open up my brain again.

One of the difficulties of being a diabetic, and a teacher is that you may upset the kids. It caught everyone out the first time it happened. I was teaching my top year 11 GCSE class – good, clever kids. I can't remember, but Mary Stuart (the Senior Mistress at the time) called the ambulance. One member of staff said later, that he was walking across the playground at break time, passing the ambulance and said to some sixteen year old girls, "Who is it?"

"Oh, it's ok Sir, it's only Mr Brookes."

Since then, the responsible kids in a class were asked to keep an eye on me in case I started to struggle in class, and if so, to run across to the office for a member of staff. Of course, you guessed it. On more than one occasion, pupils would rush for help yelling "Mr Brookes is acting weird, Sir/Miss!" when I was perfectly ok.

Mary Stuart was the school tyrant. Pupils were terrified of her, and staff similarly. I once asked her, why at break time, did she always drink her coffee standing with her back up against the wall? She smiled at me and said, "Never have your back to the enemy." Of course you could never have a joke with her – she was also an ex PE mistress. Well, not strictly true. If you're a type 1 diabetic with low blood sugar recuperating in her office. Everyone called her Mrs Stuart, but according to Barbara, who was there, I constantly called her Mary, and being a young chap as well, I gave her chat up lines, as well as winking at her.

Barbara said that since then, I was the only male she ever smiled at. Generally speaking, I was good at Branston and can't think of any other instances of misbehaviour.

The mouse incident

I think I may have been to the pub. It was a free house called the 'Plough Inn' between Potterhanworth and Bardney, at the bottom of our lane within easy walking distance and it was the only building for miles. It was heaven.

Barbara and myself were in bed – me fast asleep when Mr Mouse came out to play. Now Barbara didn't like mice – they were almost as bad as spiders. She jumped out of bed in terror and left it to me. Half asleep I was crawling on the floor at 2am trying to catch this mouse in a box. Low blood sugar and vigorous exercise don't go together. The next I remember was waking up in Lincoln County Hospital. This episode is Brookes folklore.

This is Barbara's version. It never changes, so must be true. After some time with Mr Mouse, I went back to bed and drifted away – too late for Barbara to rescue me. My twitching woke her up, so she rang the ambulance service, as I was being very uncooperative. The stairs were very steep and narrow and there was only enough room for the two big paramedics to carry a wheelchair. The wheelchair got parked by the bed, a dressing gown was put on me and I was put into the chair – still twitching.

The next part has caused years of party conversations. One paramedic tried to put my slippers on, one at a time. He knelt down, put one on and moved to the other, but my leg then performed a Georgie Best move, and the slipper flew across the room, just missing the other guy. "Look Captain, put this slipper on or we can't go." He would then put it back on, and the other flew off in the other direction. They were both calling me Captain by now, with Barbara trying to be stern with me, and laughing at the same time. This game evidently went on for a while, with me being utterly uncooperative. The slippers were still flying off in all directions as they carried me down the stairs.

Barbara was still smiling when at the hospital a small Asian doctor on night duty who's English was not perfect, asked her what happened. She launched into a graphic explanation of this mouse running around the bedroom under the dressing table and bed. A look of perplexity and confusion stopped him from asking any more questions.

The reasons for such episodes are sometimes complex and sometimes simple. The following day you can nearly always work out where it went wrong. Sometimes, the more frightening ones are where you can't identify why you've hypoed.

I do believe on occasions, insulin stores itself up in small quantities, perhaps because of a combination of foods eaten, and then releases itself. If this coincides with lowish blood sugar, you're on your way to a hypo. Usually though, you can identify the causes. In the 'Captain mouse' example, it was alcohol, along with exercise at an unusual time of day.

The Dark Side

I will give you further examples later on, but these are what I consider the most frightening part of being a type 1 diabetic. That is, slowly coming out of a coma. Some are unsettling, others are terrifying. The following is an average 'trip'.

Things are very, very black and I am scrabbling around in the dark trying to get myself out of a hole I'm in. It's like a small cave with no room to manoeuvre. I'm aware I can't make any sense of the situation I'm in. I am confused and I seem to have been here forever. I'm beginning to panic.

I realise I must be getting somewhere as I can see the odd flash and beam of light in the distance. I try to move towards the light, but I can't move, I'm still stuck. It's getting so I can hear sounds in the distance and I try to get onto my knees to crawl. It's no good. I realise that there are one or two voices I can hear, but are they coming to rescue me or to harm me? Things are terribly wet and slippery around me and I'm freezing cold. Noises are getting louder, shafts of light are flashing from one side to another and I hear more garbled voices. Have they found me? Voices are very loud and frightening now. Then someone shouts, "Paul!"

My brain kicks in and I'm out of the coma. Usually I'm on a trolley in resuscitation in A&E. A nurse has got a hold of my hand and is yelling my name. I'm wet through with sweat and freezing cold. The coldness will last for a good hour.

Another version of a trip is this. Someone finds me in a heap somewhere, but I'm in too deep to sense anything. Emergency services get to me and put a line of glucose (or equivalent) in. My blood sugar begins to rise. I can't move and feel trapped as I'm strapped down on an ambulance stretcher to control the convulsions and keep the line in. I'm wet through with sweat.

I become slowly aware of light. It could be the ambulance medic is looking into my eye for dilation observations, or the ambulance light above my head. Bringing me into A&E on a stretcher, I'm slowly becoming aware of movement. My hearing senses have heightened (I don't know why this is) and the noise and voices around me are deafening. Thank God. I'm rescued.

To the medical people out there, a plea. When you find a diabetic in an insulin coma, get them out of it as fast as you can. This may involve new drugs that can be administered fast in an ambulance that act really quickly. Bringing us out slowly is terrifying.

In 1982, Barbara and I got married. We had been living together for a number of years now, and she was fed up of being a girlfriend and not next of kin when I ended up in hospital. Protocol was such that only next of kin were given medical reports over the phone.

The next year I was promoted to Head of Maths Faculty at the Seely School in Nottinghamshire. We moved to a small village Flintham and bought a part derelict cottage that needed lots of work doing to it. I never learn.

I'm misunderstood

These are the times when the person looking after you during low blood sugars/hypos just wants to jump up from your side and yell, "Stop staring, he's not pissed, just f-----g well help me." I wonder how many diabetic's carers/friends this has happened to? Everything seems to be going swell, perhaps holding hands, looking in shop windows and then they suddenly sit down – not necessarily on a seat, just anywhere. People tend to walk around you, perhaps saying things under their breath like, "Drunk at this time of day – disgusting!"

I've done this twice in one cafe in Newark, many years ago. The first time I sat on the outside step, refusing to move. Barbara managed to get me into the cafe and sit me in a corner. I bet she wished she had a sheet she could just pop over me. The second time I was sat on the steps on the way up to the loo. Barbara says that I was again being uncooperative and people were stepping over us whilst going to the loo. How much easier it would be if someone passing just asked if help was needed? This type of situation happened numerous times with my second wife Jennifer – read on.

These incidents made us more aware of people in difficulties around us. Not far from the cafe in Newark where my blood sugar plummeted, Barbara and myself came across a frail old lady who was on her hands and knees, trying to rescue her Kentucky Fried Chicken. We tried to help but she was a carbon copy of me in a hypo. We rang for an ambulance, saying that we thought she may be diabetic. The ambulance arrived quickly and a paramedic rushed over to her. On seeing her he said, "Hello Joan. Have you been down to the Salutation again?" She was blind drunk.

I still didn't drive because of my restricted eyesight, but Penny in the next village took me to work as she went past our cottage every morning and night, as she taught Art at the same school. We all became good friends. Again, the village pub was just 200 yards away along a very minor village road. The white line down the middle was excellent for me as there was little lighting. Coming back from the pub was sometimes interesting. The white line was ok, but I often drifted past our cottage and was often going down the hill out of the village before I realised.

A few years on, perhaps around 1984, the blind eye was giving me a bit

20

of trouble. It coincided with an annual trip to Moorfields. It became very painful but I hung on until my appointment. My left eye was stable, but the right eye had an ulcer which was causing the pain. I had two choices, it was either regular injections, or removal. It was perhaps about midday when we were having this conversation. I decided to have it removed as it would only be problematic in the future.

By 2pm I was on a ward, and by early evening the operation had been done. I managed to phone Barbara late afternoon before the surgery.

I awoke around 2am with a patch over my right eye. I thought I'd gone to heaven briefly as an attractive nurse was sat by my bed holding my hand. I was intrigued by the four large black felt tip arrows drawn on my face pointing at the eye to be operated on. Evidently my left eye was covered by a large patch. No mistakes here.

I was going to be about a week in hospital according to the staff nurse. By teatime, the surgeon said that I could go home the next day. Barbara arrived by train to collect me, which turned out to be quite traumatic for her.

The train she caught was full of rugby supporters going to a big match, and all were well oiled by mid morning. They all managed to budge up to find Barbara a seat, so she sheepishly accepted.

One young supporter, holding his can of lager, turned to Barbara and said, "I know what you would like," and putting his hand into his bag, pulled out a big flask of tea. She said she felt quite safe with her new mates.

In the afternoon we made our way back. I felt quite ok – little or no pain and Barbara leading the way. I can't remember the trip back, but we arrived safely in Flintham.

Then the morphine began to wear off, leading to uncontrollable shaking and pain. I had an eye cavity, but the front of the socket had a perspex transparent lens with a hole in it wedged in to keep the eye open. A patch covered the evidence.

A local nurse popped in to see me, but sent me straight to the GP. He was more terrified than us, saying he wasn't an expert in this field. Not the sort of thing to say to Barbara. "F-----g hell, get your hands dirty then," and other similar expressions were directed to him. The drugs he prescribed me put me in fairyland for days. Alas I recovered.

The prosthesis

In only a couple of weeks time I was back at Moorfields for a quick check up. The socket was healing nicely and was still reasonably shaped. So I was sent next door to the prosthetics department. It was a bit unnerving as I remember. There were three or four seats in a row facing large mirrors, just as you would find in a hairdressers.

Off came my patch, a clean lens was put in the front of my eye that also had a hole in the centre. A nice man in a white coat (yes, it was getting spooky) with a large syringe, pumped a mixture, a bit like polyfilla, through the hole in the lens. I had to look forward. After a short period the lens and new eyeball were popped out. A bit of thumping and filing took place, and the eyeball put back. I had to look forward again and a pencil cross was put on it to line up with the pupil of my left eye.

Now this did look spooky. Looking in a mirror, my eye was all white, with a cross in the centre. I'm sure they got all the baddies' eyeballs for the Bond movies from here.

The ball was sent off to be hardened, painted (they took a picture of my left eye), and finished. After fitting, it was quite good. Not what I was expecting. It moved with my left eye a bit as it was against the muscles at the back of the eye.

It was so convincing, that when I went to the diabetics clinic in Nottingham, the leading consultant always had me in a side room with trainee doctors asking them to look at my eyes and note what they saw. Many didn't realise it was a prosthesis, just that the pupil seemed a bit unresponsive.

Whilst writing this, Barbara rang to remind me of a couple of incidents that had happened during this time.

The Twilight Zone

In our cottage (built 1834), the kitchen was lovely. Quarry tiled floor, pine sides, lots of sharp corners. On one occasion Barbara was in bed and I was up in the morning getting my breakfast. Insulin duly delivered and about to eat my cornflakes and toast. Barbara was hungry and asked for cheese on toast. Being the perfect husband, I stopped what I was doing and got the bread out. That's the last I remembered.

I came around on the kitchen floor feeling very ill. My eyebrow was cut and the doctor was there having put a couple of stitches in. Not much fuss made by me as I was down and out.

Having delivered some glucagon, the doctor left. Now I'd not felt like this before. I was on the edge of falling back into a coma for a while. Indeed I was in terror and asked Barbara to take me to the hospital. It was as if the insulin was fighting the glucagon for a good fifteen rounds. I had to eat more as this twilight zone was really frightening. Feeling terribly sick didn't help either, as I couldn't get anything to stay down. Slipping in and out of reality, going backwards and forwards the insulin and glucose were swapping dominant positions.

I suppose medically this is quite possible. Depending on what insulin you were on, the rate of absorption and the current level of your metabolism etc had concocted this terrifying cocktail. In 45 years of insulin dependence this was the only time I was truly panicking as I was conscious of my feelings.

Don't Panic

I don't really remember this one, but again Barbara did.

A very similar scenario. I ended up on the kitchen floor, and Barbara was newly armed with a glucagon pen. In the panic, she wasn't quite sure what to do with it. Alan, a friend from the next village, came up quickly. Both Alan and Barbara had discussions on what to do – Alan pointing out that if you got an air bubble in my veins it could be very dangerous.

You can visualise this, can't you. Me flat out on the floor and my wife and friend discussing the latest medical thinking. Medical debate wasn't appropriate here.

I'm not sure what happened afterwards, but I should imagine I was decorating the house again within the hour.

In 1988 Barbara and myself split up and she eventually went back to the Lake District where she spent her younger years. Don't say 'ah' yet. There's more to come.

I was divorced and working so I had a visual field test and I was able to drive again. What I did find was that night driving wasn't easy. Other vehicle headlights created a slight blur rather than a crisp image. Daylight driving was no problem at all.

Chapter Four: 38 – 55 years old (or 1989 – 2006)

I was busy at work and looking after the cottage. Not much time for anything else, but I joined a dating agency on Penny's advice. One sunny day I went down to Penny and Alan's (her husband) cottage with my list of prospective dates. Alan and myself didn't take long choosing the women in their 20s who were after a high octane relationship. Penny gave us both a stern lecture and I eventually sorted out three nice sounding ladies.

Now there isn't time here to mention the first two, but what episodes. A book in itself. The third lady I met a bit later. Jennifer, with her two little girls Leanne (9 years old) and Laura (7 years old) became the next big piece of my life.

We moved into a larger house in the village and married in 1991. Jennifer was very quiet and reserved, and so was Leanne. Laura and I were the naughty mischievous ones.

We became a family unit immediately with all the pressures of day to day life. Work, schools, holidays, teenage daughters finding themselves, and the occasional hypos.

After a long day at work and the usual meetings, I would sometimes collapse at night in front of the TV and begin to drift. The girls were so matter of fact about it. No panic or much concern. They usually carried on watching TV yelling "Mum, he's on his way." Jennifer would come in with a chocolate bar and Laura made me eat it. Problem solved.

Ignore it – if you dare

This is the big problem with being insulin dependent. If you try to live a normal life with all its ups and downs, your body doesn't like the excitement of trying to keep itself balanced. While insulin keeps type 1 diabetics alive – it's also a menace.

There were days when I would be teaching all day, using lots of energy. Others I would be in meetings for a couple of hours. Others I would be on courses or exam board meetings. I would often stay over as an examiner in hotels. Parents evenings were regular as were the stresses they usually conjured up. This brain activity burns up a lot of energy.

The body is marvellous in how it responds, but we sometimes make the job too big for it. I firmly believe that keeping a relatively active and challenging regime is what the human body needs, and was designed for. This is how the human body has developed over millennia. Go that little too far and things begin to go wrong.

Today's Lesson

The problem with most teenage and young diabetics is the body can handle abuse - sometimes for years - of too high blood sugars. Then of course something stops working. Kidneys fail, eyesight is damaged or fails completely. Circulation is restricted. But whilst they feel fine – what's the problem? The lesson comes later.

Often adult diabetics ask me for advice, and so I give it, but I also tell them that whilst they feel ok, they will carry on abusing their body. It takes a strong or frightened person to put themselves through a strict self inflicted regime which on the outside seems pointless.

The Toy Story

In my first year between Barbara and Jennifer, I rekindled my interest in railways and model railways in particular. I had a large trunk with a substantial amount of model railway 'stuff'. Out it came and off to toy fairs I went.

In a moment of weakness, Jennifer came with me, and caught the bug. It was to turn out in the long run, not very helpful.

Diabetes is one thing, but travelling to toy events most weekends, up and down the country, writing reports for the national press, writing books and maintaining a large house – as well as both of us working full time wore Jennifer out. Then there was the diabetes.

The "keep me horizontal" story

We bought a caravan as the girls were still young and went off to the Lakes. Good times were had by all – we had a ride on the Eskdale Railway, I never could convince the girls that it was exciting stuff. We even saw Thomas and the Fat Controller.

We packed up as planned and set out from Coniston for Hay-on-Wye. A long drive. We came across a hold up coming out of the Lakes. A mobile crane was jammed under a bridge. It looked as if the jib wasn't low enough. I said to Jennifer, "They ought to put it horizontal so that they can see where the gap is." Remember this bit.

We were going to Hay as Jennifer and Leanne were book worms, and I wanted to look for antiquarian maths books and some railway books.

Some considerable time later, we arrived. The girls helped by keeping out of the way and going for a walk. I set up the caravan and Jennifer unpacked. We had a meal, the girls got into their bunk beds and Jennifer and myself went to bed.

Yes – you guessed. The twitching started, Jennifer got the chocolate and Laura then fed me, interrupting my theatrical performance.

I was aware that I was in the caravan and lying on the bed, but neither completely out of it or with it. I kept repeating, "Put me horizontal so I know where the door is." This went on for a considerable amount of time. I also kept saying, "Make way for the Fat Destructor! Woo woo!" Note destructor not controller. Even Leanne got up for the show. We could never get her up so quickly at home.

Reasonably quickly I was OK. Of course, "Put me horizontal so I know where the door is," and the Fat Destructor have been quoted back to me by both Leanne and Laura years later.

This event had a subtle difference to the other episodes. Previous hypos put me well under and the process of coming out of the Dark Side was frightening. This was quite a shallow event and only used my recent memory. Indeed, I got most of the language of the crane under the bridge right, but the setting wrong. I had seen the Fat Controller the previous day.

Perhaps then, one of the first things to be compromised may be recent memory. Perhaps worthy of a bit of research by a medical student.

We bought a lot of books and the girls made sure I was laid horizontally so that I could see where the door was for the rest of the holiday.

This type of event was demonstrated at work on several occasions, whilst in the classroom. That is, the blood sugar is low, but the insulin is not making headway. I would be sometimes aware that when a child asks me a straightforward maths question, I wouldn't know the answer, or more specifically, I can't communicate. I was able to walk out of the class to the staffroom to get some supplies down me.

You can only function like this when blood sugar is low, and not on the way down even further, i.e. the level is pegged.

We had holidays abroad. Eurocamp and caravanning with the girls, Jennifer and myself stayed in hotels when the girls were older and did their own thing. No mishaps. Well, I did sit on my glasses in St. Malo once.

Eye bleeds again

Another morning and off to work. I had been promoted to Senior Teacher, so now was a member of the Senior Management Team. I was up in

Dave's office (he was Senior Management as well) and we were perhaps solving all the problems in education during break time.

"Shit," I said, and Dave looked at me and asked what was wrong. I could see blood beginning to swill in my eye.

We downed tools and had a couple of quick exchanges with other senior staff, and went off to the Queen's Medical Centre in Nottingham. After the usual long wait at the eye clinic I was eventually seen.

I then waited for the vitreous to clear itself (which usually took a couple of weeks) so that the hospital could use a laser to seal the blood vessels off.

In the past, after a couple of days I could see enough to get around and perhaps after a week it was clear. This time it was bad though. The eye just wouldn't clear. It's just like trying to see through a tank of water mixed with blood. It was constantly on the move and I had to wait for a temporary gap to see. As soon as the gap had appeared, it went again.

After nearly eight weeks, (still not back to work) the hospital were getting worried that the nutrients in the eye weren't working and they still couldn't see what was going on.

Luckily enough, a consultant down the corridor (who was based at Moorfields) had tried his hand at removing vitreous with good success. After a couple of visits, he explained that he could help.

Under a general anaesthetic, the vitreous was removed. I won't get technical, but lasers were used to break it down, probes emptied the eye, pressure was kept in the eye to keep its shape, water was put in, a bit of laser work and Bob's your uncle.

The procedure was then quite new. I went straight back to work. The scientists were quite intrigued at all of this, but Steve the caretaker was amazed at them putting water in my eye. I did say it caused problems in winter when it was freezing outside and I had to put anti-freeze in. He swallowed this hook, line and sinker for several days.

Jennifer hated hospitals, so found all this quite traumatic. I didn't realise all this at the time though. The risk of me losing my eyesight caused us both emotional stress. It was against my nature to worry too much though, I think Jennifer did my share.

Jennifer was now having to do all the driving. She coped admirably – even towing the caravan.

Loss of peripheral field

This is quite difficult to explain. My eye has had considerable laser treatment around the retina, but not too close. This causes scarring and dead tissue. This part of the eye then doesn't work.

What you don't get is tunnel vision as if you're looking down a tube and the outside edges are dark. There are parts around the outside of the eye that still pick up light but not shapes. There is no darkness at all. If it's not in front of me, I don't see it. If it's close up (e.g. walking and a curb) and below my knees, I don't see it. If it's six feet away I do.

My central vision is very good, I can see a good distance and read small print. Don't walk up beside me though, my eye sense won't pick you up. At school it was a bit awkward. I would be sat at my desk and perhaps a young pupil would be stood next to me with their book. I would have no idea they were there. The older pupils were a lot more aware and those sat in front of me would give me the nod.

Whoever invented cooker hoods want their eyes gouging out. (Just thought I'd say that.) The number of times I've taken chunks out of my head on it I've lost count of. Even people with good eyesight complain, so those with restricted vision have no chance.

Bad Girls

Laura used to sit on my right hand side when watching TV. She would carefully put her finger next to my right temple and say, "Paul.". I would turn round quickly and smack my false eye. This was hilarious to Laura. It usually ended in me chasing her and her screaming.

When in town, the girls would take my arm so that I didn't walk into anything whilst my head was up. Again, Laura would walk me into the low (two foot high) concrete bollards put around shops. Hysterical for Laura. Again it usually ended in me trying to retaliate, and with Jennifer disowning us.

Leanne was always a bit more reserved about the potential of hysterics at my expense. Perhaps it was because she was that little bit older. It was always a good laugh though to see your step-dad plummet into a hole whilst walking along a beach somewhere.

Good Girls

I tried to train them to be useful to their mum by trying to spot my blood sugar dropping. This is the 9x8 problem.

I asked the girls that if they thought my blood sugar was dropping, then ask me a question like, "What is 9x8?" No way would I produce the answer if my blood levels were down.

Unfortunately, they always asked what 9x8 was. I pointed out, that if my blood sugar was low I would perhaps try to avoid guilt by trying to get out of a question. If they asked me what 9x8 was, I would instinctively say 72 as I had remembered it from previous occasions. The knack was to ask a different question.

"How old is Mum?" may generate "72" from me. Pretty risky that, but it would catch me out.

The new prosthesis

My false eyeball had now been fitted for a considerable number of years and the muscles around the eye were not as 'toned' as before. If the eye watered and I scratched it, on a couple of occasions it has moved out of position.

Imagine a situation (this never happened though) if I was stood in front of a class of 13 year olds and I scratched my eye resulting in my eye looking in an unnatural direction. Mass panic and hysteria. The other 1200 pupils would know in days, and it would have been requested by lots of them for my party trick. Time to ask for a Mk 2 version.

The Mk 2 Eye

At this time, if you needed a prosthetic eye fitted, the eye would be surgically removed and a coral peg (very light, strong, resisting infection) stitched into the muscle at the back. As the functional eye moved, the peg in the other would follow. Additional coral would be fitted to the peg to fill the cavity. A lot lighter, thus more mobile, than a prosthetic eyeball. A false disc, imitating an eye, would fit neatly on the front.

I had one of these arrangements fitted by first separating the muscle at the back of the eye to fit a peg. This was really painful for a couple of weeks. For the last ten years I have never had to remove the disc to clean. Natural tears do the job.

It fools a lot of people as there are no gaps around the socket and looks quite natural.

I now had two spare eye balls. Not everyone's favourite trinket – except for Laura and her friend Alice who bagged one apiece.

Laura happened to keep hers in a pill box in the Welsh Dresser in the kitchen. On inviting her new boyfriend (if you call 26 years old a boy) who was on his best behaviour, he stood next to the dresser and Laura sat at the table. She asked him to look in the box, which he politely did. I forget the expletive now, but it did reflect his shock. Laura giggled and said, "That's mine." She still has it.

The Norfolk Trips

There is a dual meaning in this heading. Jennifer and myself, as the girls got older, spent weekend breaks and holidays in Norfolk. On some occasions they created trauma for Jennifer after an insulin 'trip'.

We enjoyed taking the caravan, with Jack the spaniel to Wells-next-the-Sea. Lovely walks with the dog. Unfortunately I sometimes got caught out. It was a combination of being out of routine (away from school kids) on holiday, physical exercise with the caravan, lots of walks, slight change of diet (including wine), and change of sleep patterns. I suppose I was almost asking for trouble.

I remember numerous low blood sugars, but also a couple of serious hypo's. From my point of view, I know that a hypo is not doing my brain any good long term, but I always seemed to be fighting fit very quickly after any such event. I needed the night's sleep though.

On one such occasion we were about to have dinner in the caravan. All the chores for the night had been done and I had just sat down. Jennifer was serving up and I had injected myself. All I can remember was drifting off, then awakening with a couple of ambulance men and a paramedic in the caravan. I didn't feel that bad, and a little later went to bed. That of course was not nearly half of it.

Jennifer had realised I was drifting off and tried to get some chocolate down me – to no avail. As many people perhaps experience with diabetics, there is a tendency to be uncooperative. Clenching the teeth together when trying to administer chocolate being one of them.

In my case I am perhaps thinking that I am OK and resent the intervention of someone who thinks I need help. Part of my rationality closing down.

She tried to ring for an ambulance but the signal was poor. The reception office was made aware of the problem via staff on the site and eventually the ambulance arrived all the way from Hunstanton. They set to work and I eventually came round.

Jennifer handled these situations well, but it was telling on her. There were lots of scenarios going through Jennifer's mind no doubt. Where's the hospital, how would she pack up and hitch up the caravan etc. I of course was not sharing this type of stress, but others instead.

A trip to Fakenham from Wells was something we always tried to fit in. Food market, shops, antique bookshop. On one occasion we were walking along the main street and my sugar levels were dropping. Making little sense, Jennifer hauled me into a small cafe and let the owner know the problem. Of course, I was off with the fairies by now, but luckily the woman there was either diabetic or had a relative who was diabetic. Again discreetly deposited in the corner I had light refreshment.

We left the cafe and went into town. As mentioned before, my recovery rate is very quick, and as this was a shallow hypo, my body didn't need to sleep it off. We visited an antique centre and bought a small table which I was able to carry alone. Walking back to the car I had the table upside down on top of my head as we walked past the small café that rescued me. A couple of women were looking out at me, arms folded. Jennifer swung the door open quickly and announced, "He's all right now, thanks." Whoops.

These situations are quite manageable as I am mobile and cooperative and usually unnoticed by others. Of course the hypo ones are traumatic.

Our interest in toy fairs was perhaps at a peak now. Jennifer was writing reports for a national magazine and I went along with her as the muscle (I've made myself smile). Sometimes we would also trade.

This would involve Jennifer driving, me unloading and setting up the tables whilst Jennifer walked around the event with her notebook. Most of the time this worked well – sometimes it didn't.

Getting up at 4:00am – 5:00am to drive to events, I had to watch the insulin. I usually waited until we got to the event (perhaps 8:00am ish) before taking my insulin usually sat in the car. One injection in the stomach and one in the leg. The latter involved me dropping my jeans. I'm sure this has brought some odd looks from passing lorry drivers in the past. Visualise me with my jeans down, with a syringe in my leg and Jennifer happily drinking a cup of tea.

Norfolk Showground this time. An all day toy fair, with an early start. On arrival, the insulin was injected and breakfast was eaten in the car(usually cereal and toast). No trade table this time, so both of us were walking the event before doors opened to the public. Jennifer with her notepad went off, and I wandered around looking for interesting items.

At about 9:00 the insulin started kicking in. I don't know why this time as everything seemed to be normal.

I remember walking around in a dream for some time, but I managed to sit on a chair against a wall. No ambulance was needed this time as Jennifer managed to rescue me.

Whilst I sat on the chair though I did go into violent convulsions/spasms. Quite frightening I think for the few dealers around. In a short time though I was ok.

Jennifer has since told me that she found events like this extremely stressful as she was always looking over her shoulder to see where I was and that I was ok.

On this occasion, when I had recovered we walked around together and passed a table being set up by a man and his small boy, perhaps about ten years old. He pulled his dad's arm saying, "Dad, is that the man who..." immediately stopped by his dad who smiled over at us. Whoops.

This event stays in my mind as from start to finish was a relatively short time, but my body didn't like it and so went into convulsions. This exhausted me for the rest of the day. As all type 1 diabetics know, after such an event, the body reacts with profuse sweating. My shirts are always wet through afterwards and I feel really cold.

Post hypo effect

I don't think I've mentioned this before, but after hypos or low blood sugars and when blood levels have recovered, usually very quickly in my case, my intellectuality does not suffer. I can think quickly and my sense of humour doesn't seem to leave me after the event. I am talking minutes to recover. There doesn't seem to be post event mental trauma. As soon as my blood sugar gets to about 3mmol then I'm back to normal thinking. I still have a wet shirt though.

Packing it in

I must admit, from 1998 until 2007 we really packed a lot into our lives, as I'm sure many families do.

In 1998 Leanne went to university in Plymouth to read English and so for the next three years, Jennifer and myself made long trips down there. As my driving license was now withdrawn, Jennifer had to do all the driving, sometimes with the caravan in tow and Jack the spaniel in the back. As part of our interest we also published a booklet for collectors of certain toy manufacturers' products.

In 2003 I retired early from teaching on health grounds, mostly because of my now limited eyesight. A consultant asked how I saw clearly to the back of the classroom. I said if there were any pupils at the very back, I just assumed they were guilty of some misdemeanour, and they usually were.

I had a cataract operation in my good eye (see later) and in 2005 Laura married Mark in Greece. A wonderful hot two weeks in Greece. No incidents at all, I coped with the heat very well.

We also published another two booklets based on our toy interests.

By 2006, things were motoring along quite well and we went on a journey of a lifetime trip for two weeks on the Trans Siberian Express from Moscow to Vladivostoc. Again, no incidents.

At the end of 2006 we published yet another toy booklet after a lot of trips to the south coast doing research. We were now well established in the toy collecting field and were very busy with something happening most weekends.

The cataract operation

This happened in 2004, a year or so after I retired. I had one eye and this had restricted field. Vision was deteriorating quickly as the eye lens was distorted, giving me a kind of cracked vision in places. This had been brought on early by the previous operation to remove the vitreous. Even getting around was becoming difficult.

As a car passenger, looking at a single white line down the middle of the road, looked like two converging lines to me. Imagine watching the football on the television. I couldn't work out the real ball from the impostor. On my regular visit to the eye clinic at Nottingham QMC in 2004 it was decided I needed a new lens. Because of the previous surgery and me only having one eye, any operation was serious.

It was pointed out to Jennifer and myself, that if for any reason a problem arose during the procedure then I would end up blind. Jennifer was asked if she wanted to risk this. Me being a mathematician realised that the odds were on my side it being successful, so we went ahead.

Evidently, cataract operations are quite quick, but mine took a long time as complications could rear their heads.

I remember the consultant doing the operation having all this equipment about my head whilst I was lying down. I had the local anaesthetic injected around my eye (I'm cringing at the thought of it even now) whilst it felt like my head was set up in all sorts of paraphernalia. She mentioned that if I had an itch on my nose or face, to give her quick notice and she would move the apparatus and scratch it. I've never had such service since. After nearly 50 minutes, I was done and the consultant congratulated me at keeping still for the whole length of the procedure. I do remember saying that it's quite surprising the strength you find when you're scared shitless. Leanne reminds me that the first thing I said to her after coming out of the operating theatre was, "Are you wearing stripy tights?" Since then my central vision has been superb – with the aid of glasses, and ignoring bloody cooker hoods of course.

Man's best friend

Living in the country meant that Jack the spaniel and myself spent a lot of time together. We would walk miles, particularly during the school holidays. The village is surrounded by fields, ancient footpaths, lanes and even an old Roman road. Jack was really good and never ran off.

I always made sure I had some chocolate with me just in case and had not been caught out on such walks – until now.

It was a hot summers day and we were making our way back home, walking along the edge of a field next to a dyke. Only about half a mile from the house, I suddenly began losing the strength in my legs, the usual tingling sensation, and again being unable to rationalise the situation I knelt down in the field with Jack watching and thought I'd have a snooze.

Some time later, without the usual withdrawal symptoms from the Dark Side, I came around. I was lying in the back of an ambulance, which was parked in the field next to where I had stopped. I was feeling very sick and was in fact sick. Looking out, Donna, a young mum and neighbour, was holding Jack's collar who, when he saw my movement, leapt into the back of the ambulance causing the crew to panic with all their equipment. Jack made himself comfortable across my chest. I think he sensed my slight discomfort and returned quickly to Donna who was asking him very nicely to come out of the ambulance.

Now Donna has a wonderful way with words and a unique way of expressing herself. There is no way of misunderstanding her sentiment when she gets going. It usually means trying to link up the words between the expletives.

Off I went to the hospital, without Jack, still feeling very sick.

Rewind about half an hour. Donna was walking down the lane on the other side of the field. She says she saw me lying down in the field and thought I was communing with some unknown female – not exactly her words. She knew it was me as she saw Jack lying down and watching. She spoke to another couple of women she passed on the lane and it appears as if similar sentiments were passed.

Some time later, Donna got home to her house diagonally across the field. Looking across the field, she noticed that Jack and myself had not moved. "Oh f—k," she says (she clearly remembers this) and chased across the field – she had remembered I was diabetic.

On arrival she didn't have her mobile phone, but yelled across the field to the previous two women who were walking back. Donna rang for an ambulance. It took a while evidently and several more calls from Donna. I think they may have been having problems with decoding the words between the expletives. Get here quickly was the sentiment.

On arrival the ambulance stopped next to the field, with me across the other side. It would have been a trek to walk across the field with equipment, so Donna suggested driving this ambulance across the field as it was quite flat and dry. They refused as it would be unsafe.

Now I have great admiration for the ambulance service, but they really didn't know what they were doing by taking on Donna. Moments later the ambulance was at my side.

On arrival at the hospital I was still feeling very sick and couldn't stop shaking. I was wheeled into a cubical on a stretcher and left lying down to recover with a nurse doing all the checks. I was wet through and freezing.

After a while the duty doctor whose English was quite poor arrived, but as mentioned before, my brain was now alert.

The usual questions were asked, but this one got me. "Now Paul, how long have you been unconscious for?" To which I replied, "Not sure really, as I was in a coma at the time."

I noticed the nurse who was watching turn on a broad smile, turn around and walk away. Now I know that forms have to be filled in and questions asked, but this one took the biscuit.

Jennifer arrived some time later. A bit of a shock getting home from work, Jack there and a note on the table (from Donna) saying Paul is in the hospital. Trauma for both of us again.

A few more tests were done, including one which had never happened before. Once I was up and walking, a young doctor asked me to walk along a white line on the floor. I suspect that this was a test to see if my balance and so brain function was normal.

One thing I do watch out for after all these years, is that if I end up on a glucose drip, they don't overdo it.

On occasions in the past, if hospitals felt I was struggling, for safety reasons they would keep me on a drip for a long time. Of course when I get home, my blood sugar is so high (eg 20+ mmol) trying to bring it down to a better level involves more insulin at a higher dose. Catch 22.

My theory is, get my blood sugar to about 10mmol defeats the insulin and I'm ok. Any more is overkill.

I wonder if the medical people agree, or is the problem that the insulin may still be working and so bring the blood sugar down again.

An expensive shopping trip

This type of situation happens usually when your fast acting insulin has run out, your blood sugar is low, but is not lowering any more. In my case, my blood sugar is between 2.5mmol and 3mmol. Consequently I'm in a happy, almost intoxicated mood. Not the right time to go into an expensive ladies shop in Nottingham. Picture very lovely ladies buzzing around a very smart shop, anxious to help you. I'm sat down on a very comfortable two seater settee to observe the proceedings. Jennifer wants a new suit.

I'm able to use my mobile phone, so text Laura saying, "I've spent £200." She texts back, "Tell her to keep going." I text back again, "It's 400 now." Back it comes, "Keep going gal." After nearly an hour there wasn't much change out of £1000. Jennifer looked great. I then sobered up and she still looked great.

I'm not sure what the lesson is here. I suppose activities (like spending money) that usually require consideration of the consequences are simplified. The low blood sugar again is stripping my mind of the socially learned habits.

This happened again recently (fast forward perhaps 4 years). Catching the bus back from Newark to my village, arms full of Christmas shopping and groceries, cold and tired. Strangely though I was happy and full of the joys of spring. I suspect my eye was slightly dilated which brightened everything up. On getting home my blood sugar was 2.5mmol.

The lesson to partners/carers here is that if a diabetic is being exceptionally cheerful and being generous with money, blood sugar might be low.

A very sad time

It was now Easter 2007, Jennifer and myself had just been on holiday with some friends and not suspecting a thing, Jennifer couldn't cope any more.

We had been married for 16 years and living on the edge with my diabetes. This had taken its toll on Jennifer.

We were extremely busy. Writing booklets based on our research, a large house in the country, away most weekends and Jennifer worked full time. Jennifer had met someone else, and they had fallen in love, and within a few months they were together. Some years later, as part of some email exchanges, Jennifer said:

"I couldn't cope with living on the edge of all those hypos – and fear I would sleep through one and you would die because of my failing to wake up. Spent many sleepless nights that you never knew about just waiting for you to start hypoing -"

Leanne and Laura to the rescue.

It wasn't an easy time for me and the girls were brilliant in their support. Neighbours and friends all weighed in. Jackie, whose son is diabetic, still keeps me in order. I was weighing at the time 11 stone and in two weeks was down to 9 stone. Not good for a diabetic.

I now had to relearn old skills and develop a strategy for the future.

Chapter Five: 56 years onwards (2007-)

Sleeping tablets, anti depressants, not eating properly, put me into auto pilot. I knew what I had to do, it was a case of trying to stabilise everything, including my head. Within a couple of months I was off the tablets and rediscovering my old university cooking skills – I'm quite good now. Social services sent out their teams to help me, but I was coping ok. My blood sugars stabilised. I now test my blood sugars at least every three hours during the day – even more if I'm out. I no longer have anyone to ask me what 9x8 is.

Don't say 'ah' yet – the return

The following months were traumatic as there was no rhyme or reason (I thought) why my blood sugars had a will of their own. I worked out it was my stressed state, but I couldn't work out why my body was suffering.

Then Barbara rang.

She had heard of my situation and was now widowed. I went to see her a couple of times and we talk regularly on the phone. I call her my Ex Ex Wife, but she prefers to be called my new friend.

Now, some things don't change and Barbara, again, rescued me from a hypo.

Remote Rescue

Carers of type 1 diabetics will recognise this.

Barbara rang me to see how things were going. Evidently I was quite chatty and responsive. Then I started to get a bit silly – which Barbara recognised, giving innane answers to questions. She told me to go and get some chocolate but I refused as I said I was perfectly ok. It took about 10 minutes evidently before I finally agreed to cooperate, and Barbara said she would ring back in ten minutes.

After ten minutes, Barbara rang, and I hadn't switched off the phone correctly – consequently it didn't ring. She found her old phone book and made several calls to people in my village. Either there was no response or people were otherwise engaged. As we all know, people these days are all very busy and many do not appreciate the possible outcomes for a diabetic slipping into a hypo.

Barbara doesn't panic, so imagine the response from Newark Ambulance Service getting a phone call from the Lake District to rescue a type one diabetic.

During this time I had sat at my table in the kitchen, having some chocolate and a cuppa when the doorbell rang. I opened the door and said something like "Shit – I know why you're here." It was a paramedic from Newark. He was closely followed by Penny and Alan from the next village who Barbara had got in touch with.

I felt a bit of a fraud, but it could have been a lot worse of course.

I suspect that a lot of type 1 diabetic carers have experienced this type of diabetic behaviour themselves.

Lack of cooperation and tricky car journeys

If a type 1 diabetic's blood sugar is falling below 2mmol, the conversation with them becomes silly, irrational and they become absolutely stubborn in accepting that something is wrong. Don't ask questions (9x8) as this won't work, just do something that has the outcome of sugary supplies in the mouth. You might get your finger nipped, but it will be worth it.

I've often wondered why I become awkward and unhelpful, but logically it is the blood sugar reducing and the capacity to negotiate solutions going. I never seem to realise there is a problem, so what's the fuss.

The most useful approach in my case is for someone to do something I'm not used to and that is shout at me and bully me. It's the surprise that helps for a few minutes.

Of course, if I was used to being shouted at then soft kindness might work. You get suspicious . It's doing something in a way that surprises me.

On one occasion, Jennifer and myself were returning from Brighton Racecourse caravan park after some research on the South Coast. I had been packing up the caravan and not gone many miles when joining the A27 at Falmer. I had spent many years here when I was at college so knew the roads – we ended up in Sussex University Car Park, Jennifer driving, me navigating. I got out a little bemused.

Jennifer is very passive and never shouts or swears – well I didn't think so. She jumped out of the car and yelled at me to "Get back in the bloody car," whilst apologising to someone walking past explaining that I was diabetic. I ate some chocolate unassisted.

Only recently did Jennifer inform me of anxious times she had when we were travelling. "How I used to panic whilst I was driving down the motorway when you started to fidget and mess with the door handle because you were going under and I was doing 70."

One one occasion I remember we were going to collect some model railway items we had just bought off eBay, heading down the M40 towards Marlow. Again, I was in charge of directions, which normally I was good at. We came to a large island, with clear directions on my lap. Do you think I could tell Jennifer which way to go? After a couple of circuits of the roundabout, we pulled into a leisure centre. I didn't feel stressed, but Jennifer did. We had some lunch (it was that time of day) went back to the car, and the rest of the journey was a piece of cake – which I'd just eaten. This interlude was quite brief but whilst in quite good control of myself, I could not think clearly at the time.

Whilst I have Leanne and Laura and good friends surrounding me as we all know, when the doors shut on your little house, you are on your own with the insulin. Keeping busy is my motivation.

I spent about four hours a day for almost a year writing a hardback book on toys. Even though I was unable to drive I picked myself up and went by train and bus to toy fairs and people gave me lifts. Sometimes I was able to take some of my stock and trade at events.

It's not just the diabetes of course, but also my restricted eyesight. People think I'm nuts to tackle the London Underground on my own when travelling from Newark to Sandown Park.

I have modified my behaviour a bit though. When walking through crowded areas I am forever walking into people. It's a case I think, that if you have peripheral vision and two people are converging on each other, you both subconsciously avoid each other. Not me of course. But strangely enough, the person I walk into almost always apologises for walking into me. At first I would apologise myself saying it was undoubtedly me, but then I got bored. It's now surprising how many people apologise to me whilst I navigate the London Underground. I now just smile and accept their kind words.

One thing you must do when you're in a situation like mine is to believe that the great British public just love to help people who are struggling.

On one occasion I got on the Tube at Kings Cross and couldn't make out the route map above the windows. I was too far away, bright fluorescent lights, and the train packed. I asked very politely, a very tall, large black guy stood next to me if he could help me read the map. Not only did he tell me how many stops I needed to go, he moved everyone out of the way when I got there with a loud booming voice. Two young teenage girls took my arms and pulled me through. I now look for crowded tube trains.

The serious point here is to have the courage to ask for help. Over the last three years I have convinced myself that I'm a quick thinking problem solver needing to do things. My eyesight lets me down occasionally and so if I'm struggling, I ask. It's not being weak about something, it's being practical.

Being on my own

After 45 years on insulin, the last three years is the longest period I've spent living on my own. You don't set out to meet someone so that later they fulfil a carer's role. I'm an old fashioned romantic really with all that it entails.

Because of how Jennifer struggled I have promised myself to regain the independence I had as a young man.

Being practical though, things are more risky now. Sleeping alone means there is no one to bail you out if you slip into a hypo when you're asleep. In the last three years this has happened to me four times. Statistically a very rare event. But of course, you only need one bad one. My liver has bailed me out on these four occasions though.

In addition, my brain seems to now negotiate with me how to best get out of an overnight hypo when I eventually come round.. It's never happened before, but I spend time working things out and developing the strategy. I don't panic, even though my body is incapacitated.

The sicky hypo

The bit that can catch type 1 diabetics out is not only how much insulin you take, but also what you eat.

It sounds a bit obvious to the medical people out there, but it's easy to come unstuck. Imagine taking your usual insulin at 6pm for your evening meal. A combination of fast and slow absorbing carbohydrate is ideal. If you take a majority of slow acting carbohydrate, you are in danger of the insulin taking over before the carbohydrate is digested. Sounds good. Unfortunately I think there may be other factors at work. What have you been doing during the day, physical exercise, sitting down, driving? A blood sugar of 8mmol at 6pm is unhelpful knowledge if you don't know how fast your body is going to absorb the carbohydrate. You could end up hypoing at 2am or have an mmol of 15 when you get up in the morning. I'm not much help here, but you just experiment with food on your body. This hypo I became aware of at about 2am, rolling out of bed and being violently sick. Almost immediately again at the foot of the bed. I spend a very long time sat on the loo having severe problems both ends. Cold, shaking and feeling terrible.

Food seemed to be the problem. I can't remember now what I ate, but it wasn't digesting very well. Suffice to say, I recovered and the only long term damage was to the carpet. Oh, and my slippers.

The Cyberman

It was dark and quiet but the Cyberman's eyes were piercing my brain. It didn't matter what I did or where I looked, he was facing me down. It was frighteningly dark with his eyes only feet away from me, he wasn't saying anything, just watching me. I began to sweat as I made out his eyes were bright blue on a black background and finally the fear subsided as I began to move and work out my exit strategy. The pressure was off for a few seconds as I reached out and switched on the bedside light. Bloody digital clock with illuminated square digits. Blood level 2.5mmol. Cup of tea and a biscuit at 3am scared him off.

As I am writing these down, it is quite apparent that different levels of blood sugar, below 4mmol, present different types of physical and mental reactions. As the mental facilities close down the diabetic falls from security to confusion to different levels of coma and nightmares.

A trip to the dark side

It's very cold and black again, no faint light at all and no sound. I'm jammed hard between the rocks of this freezing cave. I struggle but it's no good, I can't move. My head is jammed hard and I struggle to move. There's no sound or light and I continue to struggle.

After an eternity my senses begin to sharpen and there is some background fuzzy light somewhere, but I'm still jammed and there's no sound. I'm more conscious of my efforts to work myself free, and beginning to find rocks to put my hands against and push. My legs are jammed behind me, but I get a foothold. I can wriggle my head loose from between the rocks and push myself away. There's more light now. I think I'm free.

Back from the dark side. Somehow I managed to get upstairs to the bathroom whilst nearly unconscious, and fell on the tiled floor getting my head stuck between the U-bend of the toilet and the wall. My shoulders were jammed as well.

The bathroom lights were on, but I couldn't really see until I wriggled back. I sat myself down for twenty minutes with a towel around me as all my clothes were wet through with sweat. Strangely I felt reasonably ok, except for being exhausted. I boosted my blood sugar and had a cuppa. I managed a shower. Checked my blood again and went to bed.

I suppose I could call this quite a severe hypo as I went to the dark side again, but found some glucose in my liver to bring me round. On this occasion I wasn't sick and my body strength recovered quickly. It could have been worse.

Wide eyed and legless

This was a strange one. I can't recollect going to the dark side, but if so, it was brief. I was wet with sweat, I'd been sick, and found myself sat on the bottom set of the stairs. It would appear that this was a shallow hypo, but things were slightly different.

Very quickly my senses and brain were switched on. I felt as if I was ok, but knew I needed something to eat quickly to prevent a possible relapse. The solution was in the kitchen. Six metres along the hallway to the kitchen, turn left then two metres across the kitchen to the biscuits. Easier said than done.

I was quite clear headed now, but my legs wouldn't work. I thought, "Shit – stroke," - but I was clear headed and it was only my legs not working at this stage. Chest, arms and both sides appeared ok.

Time was of the essence I thought so I began to crawl a bit unsteadily towards the kitchen, but toppled over when trying to turn the corner. Again, my brain was perfectly ok and I was feeling ok as I knew I had time because my head was clear. I rounded the corner on my knees and sat down on the floor with my back to the wall, looking at the cupboard opposite at floor level.

I must be ok as I remembered my humour was intact as I told the cupboard, "Don't bloody move." It took perhaps five minutes for me to recover enough to attempt the crossing. I made it. Ate some biscuits and opened a can of Diet Coke (have to watch the waistline) and sat on the floor with my back to the cupboard.

It would be ten minutes before I attempted to stand up, leaning on the kitchen side. I wobbled badly so eased myself back down again.

It wasn't long before I was up and mobile again.

What I can't explain in this case is that I obviously had a hypo, my brain kicked in very quickly to the extent I was working out strategies to get to the kitchen, but my legs refused to cooperate.

I think that my body works on a sliding scale of mmol levels to which I can tie the loss (or gain) of certain mental and/or physical attributes, rather than all going simultaneously.

This would tie up with the brain losing the use of distinctive parts that control distinctive features, as they lose their energy.

Thinking back, it could also be that sometimes my inability to move in the cave on the Dark Side is not only paramedic straps, but the severe loss of muscle strength in my legs.

The poor bus driver

I think this was about November 2009. I was fully up and running and I needed to go to Newark to buy some bits and pieces for a toy restoration project. No problem, the Newark to Nottingham bus goes through my village, one of a nice, newish single decker fleet. I needed some acrylic paint and a rod of piano wire (don't ask).

It was a bit cold waiting for the bus in Newark, I had my woolly hat on, gloves, parka type coat, rucksack on back (containing chocolate, insulin and blood test gear) and piano wire stood against me. I got on the bus and the sun began to shine through the November cold. It was nice and warm on the bus. I thought, how cosy, and made myself comfortable. Change channel.

Dark and cold, I was struggling in a frightening cave somewhere. Only briefly, but no less terrifying. Lights began to flicker and voices got louder. Awake quickly, it took seconds to realise I was in the back of an ambulance. Two ambulance paramedics were there. One manipulating the drip in my arm and testing blood levels, the other filling in forms.

I felt awful. Freezing cold, wet through and shaking. Evidently I had drifted off, passed through my village and was discovered at the end of the journey in Nottingham, slumped in my seat. Passengers had disembarked, a queue ready to embark and a young bus driver who had only been in the job a few weeks, wanting the earth to open. He called for an ambulance instead, which parked behind the bus. Off went the bus, late of course, and I was lifted into the ambulance.

After 15 minutes or so my blood sugar was high enough for me to think about making my way home.

This episode, whilst always traumatic, wasn't as severe as those at home on my own. I was picked up quite quickly (it was perhaps half an hour at the most before I was discovered) and so the dark side didn't get its teeth into me for long, as the glucose got to work quickly.

I still felt very ill though. It was perhaps that usually after such episodes I can get warm and sleep it off.

Wanting to sort myself out I asked the guys where my hat, gloves and glasses were. "What?" they asked. All they had was my rucksack. I was now in the middle of Nottingham, stood next to the ambulance and said to myself, "Taxi." Then a bus turned up, so I realised this was the quickest way back home. I waited for everyone else to get on and showed my pass. Now this was an older driver, always pleasant and cheerful. He looked at me and said, "Are you the guy that..." My defences were down. The bus was quite full and he said, "You, sit where I can see you." A young woman near the front jumped out of her seat quickly and let me sit down.

There I sat for one of the longest journeys I've ever had. Bus lurching from side to side, up and down, with me feeling cold, wet and sick. Now the main road cuts through the village where I live, in two. The main village on the right hand side and where I live is on the left. The bus driver not only stopped the bus at my stop, he jumped out of his seat, picked me up out of the seat and said, "Right. I'll take you across the road." I said, "I'd rather stay this side please, as I live up here." He smiled.

The lady who gave up her 1 seat for me got off at this stop and said she would look after me and we walked home arm in arm. In other circumstances I would have been a very happy chappy. The problem here, as mentioned before, I was struggling badly to continue as normal after a hypo.

A rule of thumb here. After hypos, diabetics need to sleep it off, or at least lie down and rest, to let the body recover. All energy has been drained.

I rang the bus company later that day, and the nice lady rang the first driver, who had passed on the bus to another, who then got passengers to look on the floor.

The next day, I met a different driver who stopped his bus at my village stop at an agreed time. He had my hat, gloves and glasses that had been found on the floor. "Is this yours?" he said, handing over the piano wire. Aren't people caring and helpful. The model railway signal cabin, with its new handrail going all the way round (piano wire!) and me, are both fully restored.

Chapter Six: – Conclusion

The Brookes mmol sliding scale theory

I'm trying here to give a visual scale of mmol (blood sugar) levels that is particular to me. Different diabetics will have a different sliding scale, but will no doubt contain the same ingredients.
At all of these levels, your blood sugar can stick at a particular point for some time – the insulin has run out and lost its effect. The liver then gives out some glucose and you slowly recover.
The worst scenario of course is if the blood sugar keeps falling.

4mmol

This is a safe level for me. All senses very alert, but I don't want it to go lower, as a change of activity (or stress) reduces it quite quickly.

3mmol

I act quite normally, but am getting more carefree and unguarded.

2.5mmol

My rationality begins to struggle. Become happy and silly. If challenged, I can become awkward or aggressive.

2.0 mmol

My problem solving skills are suspended (can't write cheque or read a map).

1.75 mmol

I become more uncooperative, losing any learned social skill. I appear drunk. Can't help myself now.

The Twilight Zone – In and Out of Reality. I'm panicking now, I can't effect a recovery.

1 – 1.5mmol

I lose consciousness.
A trip to the Dark Side.
I shut down and have nightmares. These can be of different degrees.
A quick exit (ambulance/paramedics) reduces the scary bit, but you are usually physically drained on recovery. A long visit is very frightening. Avoid at all costs the Dark Side.
It is possible that the nightmares kick in when the blood sugar is rising. I may move from shut down to slow recovery of senses (hearing, awareness of light) through this nightmare phase. Get me out of this
impasse as quickly as possible.

Some thoughts

Being on insulin for 45 years seems very challenging to most people – but it is better than being dead! Different diabetics will see it in different ways and will either ignore it, or become a slave to insulin.
If you ignore it and let your body cope with years of abuse whilst feeling ok, you will eventually come unstuck. I know young diabetics who have had legs amputated, as circulation diminishes. I know diabetics whose sight has significantly been affected. (Oh, that's me.) Don't ignore it.
Yes, I know diabetics will face this in different ways. Some get very depressed, others will find the strength and drive from family and friends to lead a full life.
I retired early but still got in 33 years of teaching, and everything that it entails. Family and friends make my life as happy as anyone else's.
Some diabetics will find this difficult, but families can help if they understand the situations that I've tried to outline. The stress on partners can be enormous, depending on their very own nature. Some will handle it like water off a ducks back, others will at times not have the emotional resources to cope.
It is possible that a partner becomes so depressed and/or anxious about

their responsibilities that they become a distinct liability, or even hazard to the diabetic when in a hypo situation. Decisive and correct appraisals need to be made and acted upon in these situations. Seek help if you're floundering – there is plenty out there. Start with your GP.

To be defeated by the traumatic situation and walk away is a distinct possibility. Carers or partners sometimes need as much help as the diabetic. It's a team challenge.

For the diabetic themselves it is an extremely lonely time when the insulin saps your strength. You keep wanting to beat it, but there's no escape. My view is that it's playing games with me on occasion and I have to try to protect myself and win. The Dark Side is evil and frightening, but can be successfully handled.

Having just read this in one go, it sounds like hard work in places, but I have just described 45 years on insulin. If you stretch all these events out over 45 years then life is fairly normal. I spend weeks living on my own now with little or no insulin episodes. My humour is intact, but so are my coping strategies. I travel the country following my hobby and seeing friends. It is very important not to lock yourself away – go for it.

A quote from Jennifer sticks in my mind. "You're dead a long time."

Here's to the next 45 years – well, I'll at least try.

Postscript

When I started this project I precisely stated the start date as 1965. It is now January 2011 and the first draft is finished.

No doubt, further things will happen in the future that may be worthy of some thought, but I'll do something else for a while now.

I finished the draft last night and was in bed by 11pm, blood mmol was 7.0. At 2am, I was wet with sweat and thought, "Here we go." I made a cuppa and tested my blood – it was 8.2mmol. "Strange," I thought. It's not the insulin.

Could it be I've had a sympathetic menopausal event, or just any other normal event, cold, virus etc. At 3am I started thinking.

My body has been reacting to insulin for 45 years. Messages are sent from my brain to my body, telling it to sweat under certain circumstances.

I wonder if it is possible for these well established routes to be stimulated by things other than just insulin. Interconnected facets of the brain may stimulate these well trodden portals to open. In other words, because of long term use of insulin, my body can perhaps mimic insulin driven outcomes.

Now there's a thought.

Paul Brookes
mastermodels@btinternet.com